UNCLOG YOUR ARTERIES
How I Beat Atherosclerosis

By

Gene McDougall

ISBN: 0-75962-279-5

This book is printed on acid free paper.

1stBooks - rev. 7/25/01

"Change your thoughts and you change your world."

- Norman Vincent Peale

CONTENTS

Preface
What your heart surgeon won't tell you.

If you're anything like me, you are not physically or emotionally ready to do the research necessary to make an informed decision when you have just had a heart attack and are told that you need bypass surgery. Your heart surgeon should be sure that you have a thorough understanding of your options and their individual ramifications before consenting to the operation. For instance, you should know that half of all bypass grafts close within five years. Not all heart surgeons will tell you this.

I wish there had been a book that told me concisely, in easy to understand language, what I wanted to know about my condition and the various options open to me – a "how-to" manual to help me beat the odds. To my knowledge, no such book existed.

So after my surgery, I did the research and wrote the book myself. Now that it exists, you won't have to spend countless hours, even years, poring through volumes of information about a variety of subjects such as vitamins and minerals, prescription medication, exercise, stress, nutrition, blood tests, stress tests and weight control as well as health insurance and Medicare paperwork. I have put it all together for you in one book with no long-winded medical double-talk to wade through. Just the basic, need-to-know stuff, told in plain, everyday English.

This is the survival manual I needed but could not find when I had my heart attack in 1986. Since I had made it my business to learn all I could about my condition after my bypass surgery, I was ready when my bypass grafts started to close just four years later. Using the methods described in this book, I actually reversed the process! As a result, I have enjoyed a wonderfully healthy, active life ever since. I hope my story will help others achieve the same happy results.

1. MY HEART ATTACK

It was June 6, 1986, and I was enjoying a restful Sunday at home. Suddenly I began to sweat profusely, then became nauseated and started vomiting. I took my blood pressure. Usually at the high range of normal, it was now alarmingly low - 83 over 63. I called my doctor. He told me to get to the emergency ward of the hospital at once. Soon after my arrival there, I was told it was a heart attack. I could not believe it.

In spite of my insistence that I was okay (it was now three hours after the attack and I felt fine), I was wheeled up to coronary intensive care where I spent the next few days. After that, I was closely monitored on the cardiac floor another six days. I was then sent home to rest three weeks before returning for an angiogram - a procedure involving the insertion of a catheter into an artery and on into the heart. Dye is then injected into the catheter and monitored on a TV

1

screen to see if it runs into any blockages. Rather than resulting in a clean bill of health as I had expected, the angiogram showed the right main artery completely blocked and the other main arteries 75% to 95% blocked. Two weeks later I consented to bypass surgery (quintuple, as it turned out), an option I might not have agreed to if I had known then what I know now.

How had it come to this? Although I was 57 years old, I had stayed in shape by playing two hours of vigorous tennis at least three times a week for the past 15 years, had not smoked for 22 years, almost never touched alcohol and stayed away from salt, sugar and eggs. I did not consider myself overweight, and my blood pressure was normal with medication.

I did not want another heart attack and I certainly did not want any more open-heart surgery, which meant some questions would have to be addressed:

1. What could I do to reduce the stress that I knew had been a key factor in my heart attack?

2. Was I exercising properly?

3. Were my eating habits really as healthy as I had believed?

4. What medications would be best for me?

This project now became my number one priority, and has resulted in my learning more than I ever expected to know about the heart, the body and the enormous power of the human mind and spirit. I feel lucky, not only for having survived the heart attack, but for having had it in the first place. Why? Because nothing short of such a traumatic event could have shocked me into finally taking a hard look at myself and then making the changes that were not only necessary but long overdue.

I began a journal, posting every change in my medications, diet and lifestyle from that point on - also listing each significant event in the years leading up to

Gene McDougall

the heart attack. This cause-and-effect experiment did not yield immediate results. In fact, a setback occurred in 1990 when my annual stress test revealed an abnormality. A thallium stress test was then ordered, which showed that my grafts were beginning to close after only four years. A thallium stress test is similar to a regular treadmill stress test, except that at peak exertion, thallium is injected into a vein. Exercise is then stopped and the patient lies on a table under a scanning camera. By now the thallium has reached the heart, so the camera can take a series of pictures measuring the percentage of heart muscle not receiving adequate oxygen. If an area of the heart muscle is receiving an insufficient blood supply, it will show up as a dark area or "cold spot". After a few hours, more pictures are taken, and if the blood flow deficit (cold spot) has filled in (or "redistributed"), the muscle cells are not dead and the condition is reversible if blood flow to the area can be increased.

My 60 percent cold spot in February of 1990 was reduced to only 10 percent in December of 1992 - a dramatic improvement in just 34 months. It is not clear whether the improved blood flow is the result of clogged arteries unclogging, new collateral circulation developing, or both - but my heart and I don't care. We're happy.

I have charted each and every significant change I made during this period as new studies in the field were published and I acquired a greater understanding of my own condition. These charts appears later in this report. I cannot be sure precisely which changes had the most effect in this turnaround, or whether some had no effect at all - but I feel that some conclusions, which I will enumerate later, can safely be drawn. One thing I know - I will stick with my current lifestyle and continue my present diet, medications and vitamin therapy because the combination of some or all of those things has restored

5

Gene McDougall

me to the robust good health that only a few years ago was in serious jeopardy.

I was extremely fortunate that my heart attack caused no significant damage to the heart muscle. It would probably have been fatal if my years of tennis had not caused my body to build a strong life-saving system of collateral circulation. This served as a natural bypass, supplying my heart with the blood it needed when my main artery closed.

In July of 1992, six years after my heart attack and bypass surgery, I won a gold medal in tennis at the Minnesota Senior Olympics, playing three matches in one day for a combined total of four and a half hours. I won the final match when, after splitting the first two sets (both were tie-breakers), my opponent was unable to continue. To me, this was pretty convincing evidence that my heart was getting an ample supply of blood.

Even now, more than a decade after my heart attack and bypass surgery, I play one or two hours of singles tennis several times a week. Although my opponents are usually younger than I am, I get a great deal of satisfaction from knowing that if one of us runs out of gas, it won't be me.

Now let's get into the four categories identified earlier as problems needing my attention. Since I believe stress was the precipitating factor in my heart attack, we'll start there.

2. STRESS

You are bound to feel stress if you are not in control of the things in your life that matter the most, and I believe a man's work and his love life are at the top of the list. If both of these are in bad shape, his emotional and physical well-being are in serious jeopardy.

I had a job I loved until 1981, when my immediate superior, whom I liked and respected, retired. He was replaced by a man I held beneath contempt both as a manager and as a person. I will go into no more detail except to say that my 1986 heart attack should not have come as a surprise. Fortunately for me, our company was taken over by a larger one during that period, and shortly thereafter (in 1987) a generous early retirement package was offered to those of us who were old enough and had enough years of service. It was perfect! I was 57 years old with 31 years of service. I jumped at the chance, as did just about everyone else who qualified.

But even after my heart attack and bypass surgery, and fully realizing that I would be retired in six months, I continued to be consumed by the rage that had been building inside me. Knowing that I could not continue like this without inviting another heart attack, I went to the Immanuel Medical Center in Omaha in December of 1986, where I underwent a two-day evaluation in their Stress and Preventive Medicine program. I was found to have all the type A characteristics including competitiveness, perfectionism, a sense of time urgency and a chronic state of vigilance. I also scored very high in anxiety, depression and hostility - in fact the highest they had ever seen! It was recommended that I see a psychologist in my local area who was knowledgeable in the field of stress and hostility. I did so and benefited greatly, but it was not a quick fix. Although it involved many gut-wrenching months of soul-searching, I urge anyone in need of such help to admit it and lose no time in finding a good therapist.

While it is not uncommon to be emotionally confused and hard to live with following bypass surgery, I probably abused the privilege because it took me so long to let go of my anger over the way my work environment had been destroyed. This put so much strain on my marriage that finally, in October of 1990, my wife and I separated. Even though we are each now happily following the beat of our own drummers, we remain close, caring and supportive. In fact, we have become good friends and enjoy every Christmas season together in sunny Arizona where she now lives. In many respects our relationship is better now than at any time in our 37 years of marriage.

In my opinion, no discussion of affairs of the heart would be complete without a few words about dogs. Gerne, the beautiful miniature dachshund who brightened my life from 1981 to 1990, made it abundantly clear to me each and every day that she truly loved me with all her heart, and I felt the same way about her. We did not find each other until she was eight years old so we only had a few good healthy years together, but even in her later years when she was blind and deaf she was a great source of happiness. During the last two of her 17 years of life she could not tell us when she had to answer the call of nature, so I would sleep with her in my arms all night long. About every two hours she would begin to fidget, automatically waking me up so I could take her out. But finally, when she became arthritic and so sensitive to sunlight that she would jerk her head in pain when she went out into the sunlight, we had to do the unthinkable and let her go. The vet agreed to let me hold her as he injected the shot, so she died peacefully knowing only that she was contentedly falling asleep in my arms with her ears being stroked, a daily ritual we had enjoyed together so many times before.

I cried for weeks, and even after all this time, the tears are welling up again as I write these words But looking back on the wonderful years we had together, I know it was all worth it. This I can promise - you will never feel lonely or unloved if you have a Gerne in your life.

Another aspect of life that can affect your emotional health is the management of money. I have finally come to realize that it is folly to try to "get rich quick." Every time I have tried, it has taken me years to recoup. I am too ashamed to tell you how many thousands of dollars I have squandered in commodity futures, stocks, options and limited partnerships. Do not - I repeat - DO NOT try to get rich in a hurry. That is just another form of gambling. If a few thousand dollars more or less would not change your lifestyle, why bother? The stress is simply not worth it. And if a few thousand dollars more or less WOULD change your lifestyle, then gambling in any form is something you simply cannot afford, either financially or emotionally. DON'T DO IT!

Of course you can't just stick your money under your mattress (although that would be preferable to buying stock options or commodity futures), so what should you do? After many years of expensive lessons in the school of hard knocks, my financial game plan has evolved into a simple one. I invest in mutual funds only. Too many bad things can happen to an individual company, and its stock price is too easily manipulated by professionals. Even when you pick a winner, knowing when to sell is almost impossible. A few years ago I sold Amgen for a small profit, whereupon it promptly tripled. So, even when you make a profit, you can have regrets. The emotional roller coaster of individual stock buying and selling is not for me, and if you want peace of mind, consider the possibility that it may not be for you either.

Nice profits can be made with mutual funds. I have brokerage and money market accounts with both

Charles Schwab and Fidelity through which I do all my checking and purchase all the funds I want - most with no loads, commissions or fees. It is even possible to buy some funds which have been closed to new investors, since any broker currently handling a fund is carried on the fund's books as a shareholder, and is therefore entitled to purchase additional shares (in this case, for resale to you, the client). Some funds have closed this loophole, so if the fund you want is closed to new investors, this may or may not work - but it's worth a try. The toll-free numbers for Schwab and Fidelity are (800) 785-7977 and (800) FIDELITY respectively. By the way, if you have a computer, a wonderful free source of excellent investment information is The Motley Fool. Just log onto Fool.com.

Having said this, I must confess to holding small positions in half a dozen stocks at the present time - just for fun, with money I have already written off as entertainment expenses. I found one of the most exciting stocks I ever owned as a result of the research I was doing on coronary artery disease. It was PLC Systems, and when I discovered it in 1993, I filed it away under "future possibilities". It was a new company which was working on an alternative to bypass surgery, improving blood flow to the heart by using laser beams to drill 30 or so microscopic holes in the heart itself rather that by grafting bypass veins. Since this could be done without splitting open the chest and stopping the heart, the concept sounded exciting - but it was still experimental. Then, in April of 1995, I ran across an item in the local paper announcing that this new procedure, called transmyocardial revascularization (or TMR), was being applied successfully in a number of hospitals, including one right here in the Chicago area. I bought some stock right away and called the company to make sure I was put on their shareholders list to receive information about their progress on an ongoing basis. In December of that same year, their patented Heart

Laser technology was declared to be no longer experimental, making it eligible for Medicare coverage. It was good to know there was now another alternative to bypass surgery. Luckily, I sold the stock for a 400% profit after holding it for just under one year. I say "luckily" because not long after that, they ran into patent trouble and there were even some accusations involving stock manipulation. In fact, PLC is currently the defendant in a class action lawsuit. As I said, stocks are a dangerous game.

Hobbies are another good way to overcome stress. My playing tennis pays off in a number of ways. Not only is it fun, but it is also good exercise and provides me with a great network of friends.

Another hobby I enjoy is what I'm doing now - writing. It is especially fulfilling to write a "how-to" piece, because while you are helping others, you are also increasing your own knowledge as you collect, sort and organize information on the subject you have chosen. While you should write about something you are involved in, care about or perhaps do better than the average person, by no means do you need to be an expert in the field. If your experience or research makes you more knowledgeable than the average person, this means there are millions of people out there who know less than you do about the subject and can therefore benefit from what you have to say.

It is really fun to write your book, report, article or story on a computer or word processor. What a pleasure it is to type your first draft knowing that later on, you can effortlessly insert, delete or change words, phrases or paragraphs anywhere in the text. Not only that, but when you are done, the computer will go through the entire manuscript finding and correcting all your spelling errors. If you are computer illiterate, learning how to use one can be an absorbing and rewarding hobby in and of itself. I don't know what I would do without my e-mail and the vast information resources available on the internet.

Gene McDougall

Exercise, sex, laughter and an upbeat, optimistic attitude cause the brain to release endorphins into the system. These wonderful little critters relieve stress and possess supernatural healing qualities. If you want to be convinced, read Norman Cousins' "Anatomy of an Illness", "The Healing Heart" and "Head First".

Years ago, I taped a segment of one of the "Bloopers" TV programs showing Steve Allen breaking up while trying to do a bit on his late night show. I have played it back dozens of times over the years, and tears of laughter still roll down my cheeks whenever I watch it. At such times, I can almost feel the endorphins frolicking inside my body.

It is important to recognize that sex is not only your birthright; it is the birthright of every living thing. Insects, as incredibly unattractive as they are, have sex. Even trees, in spite of their obvious limitations, manage to do it. It is an enormously popular activity, so if your mother told you sex was naughty and disgusting, get over it. You were misinformed. This is definitely something you don't want to miss out on. Trust me.

To get back to laughter for a moment, I consider myself lucky that I can see humor in almost everything. In fact, sometimes an incident that would go almost unnoticed by most people can cause me to laugh uncontrollably. Let me relate one such incident that, although it happened circa 1960, still flashes into my consciousness now and then, sending me into spasms of laughter.

I was in downtown Marshalltown, Iowa on a business trip, and while walking down the sidewalk I saw an old man in overalls walking in my direction. He was about a block away when we first noticed each other. Both of us were immediately aware that we were on a collision course, so we simultaneously changed course - him to his right and me to my left, which of course resulted in our still being headed straight at each other As the distance between us rapidly shrank, we made several more adjustments, each a little more frantic but all of them canceling each other out. At the last possible second, our adjustments narrowly averted a head-on collision, and as we brushed by each other I heard him mutter, "Jesus Christ." He then disappeared behind me as we continued on our separate ways. I never looked back and never saw him again, but I can't help thinking about our encounter now and then. Not funny? Sorry. Maybe you had to be there. (Damn - I'm starting to giggle again.)

Before we leave the subject of humor, I can't resist plugging the book I co-authored with my friend, Nelson Campbell. It's called "Cow Pies, A Messy Journey Through the Pasture of Life." a collection of whimsical letters we wrote to each other over the previous 12 years, using fictional names such as "The Venerable Reverend Elton Jones," "Uncle Randy, Advisor to the Wretched," and "Reverend Clarence Klotz." A sample letter follows. If you think you would enjoy 228 pages of this sort of thing, send a check for $11.95 to me at 2811 Bel Aire Drive, Arlington Heights, IL 60004 and I'll send you a copy. What the heck, I'll even pay the postage. If you decide you want one, don't wait too long. Only a few hundred were printed, so they are fast becoming collector's items. But be forewarned - if you are a member of the right-wing Christian Coalition and can't laugh at yourself, save your money. You will not be amused.

Dear Clarence,

As I sit here in solitary gloom listening to my arteries harden and my body deteriorate, an overpowering feeling of despair engulfs me. Do I have time left to turn my life into something that will allow me to die a happy and fulfilled man?

I think so.

Little by little, my unrealized dreams, missed opportunities and outright failures have provided me with a wealth of experience to draw upon as I put together my exciting new business plan. This time, I have a winner if there ever was one. Forget the door-to-door breast exam service, the mom and pop fire station – forget all the traditional thinking that has held me back in the past. I have transcended all that and am now thinking outside the box. Hold on to your hat. Are you ready? I intend to form a not-for-profit religious organization! Ninety percent of the money taken in will be paid to me in salary and bonuses, with 10% going to the various charities that we will support. Do you see the beauty in this? The Elton Jones Charity Foundation (EJCF) will need to do no heavy lifting, as it were (no hands-on work among the poor, the diseased or the otherwise distasteful). All EJCF need do is select which charities to donate 10 percent of our income to, and feather our nest with what is left.

I would not have told you all this if I could not find a way for you to share in the profits. I am pleased at this time to offer you the position of Chief Charity Selector (CCS) of EJCF. You will be in charge of the entire 10% of total EJCF income earmarked for charity, with the responsibility of choosing which charities are selected to receive our money. Half of this amount goes into your pocket as compensation for your services. At first glance, this may not seem like much, but don't forget that we haven't factored in the kickbacks to you from the charities vying for our handouts. Make no mistake – we're talking big money here, brother!

And here's the grabber. As men of the cloth running a not-for-profit organization, we will never pay a dime in taxes! Is this a great country or what? To seal the deal, I am prepared to offer you the other half of your 10% budget to run the media operation necessary to produce our income. After some number crunching, this appears to leave nothing for the charities, but we can work that out later. The important thing is to get started ASAFP.

Praise the Lord,

Elton

Gene McDougall

3. EXERCISE

By now you know that my main source of exercise is tennis. In fact, that is just about my only form of exercise. There is some disagreement about whether tennis is an aerobic or anaerobic activity, so let's start out by defining both terms. If the exercise is light, moderate or isometric (short, intense burst of activity), that is considered to be anaerobic exercise and is of little use in improving cardiovascular fitness. It is only when you cross the "anaerobic threshold" from moderate to more intense activity that you are beginning to exercise aerobically. Aerobic exercise improves your cardiovascular health by increasing the efficiency with which your body uses oxygen for energy.

To be sure your exercise is providing you with the cardiovascular benefits you seek, it is necessary to get your heart beating fast enough to achieve your target heart rate and keep it there for at least 20 minutes.

24

This should be done at least three times a week. To find out what your target heart rate is, you must first determine your maximum heart rate. You can do this by subtracting your age from 220. Your target heart rate is 60 to 80 percent of this maximum rate. For example, if you were 65 years old, your maximum heart rate would be 155 (220 minus 65). To reach your target heart rate, you would therefore need to get your heart pumping at between 93 and 124 beats a minute (60 to 80 percent of 155). Check your pulse on the inside of your wrist for 15 seconds and multiply by four.

After learning this formula, I checked my pulse the first few times I played, but after I was satisfied that I was reaching my target heart rate, I no longer bothered. Generally, I am satisfied that my exercise is aerobic if I am sweating. By the way, the more fit you become, the more exercise it will require for you to get your heart beating fast enough to reach your target heart rate.

For me, singles tennis is aerobic because I depend on hustle rather than skill. I don't hit the ball hard enough to end many points with outright winners, so I must try to keep the ball in play until my opponent makes a mistake. This can result in very long and strenuous points, so the heart rate stays right up there as long as there is not a lot of time wasted between points or games. As a diabetic, the more vigorous forms of exercise are the most beneficial to me because that is when the body will begin to burn carbohydrates (glucose, or blood sugar) as fuel. Of course, once in a while I will find myself playing a tournament match with some old guy who wants to sit down between every other game, which pretty much destroys any aerobic benefits that could otherwise have accrued to either of us.

One caveat about tennis or any competitive sport. If you find yourself arguing about line calls, cursing at yourself when you miss a shot or getting depressed when you lose, you are what I call a "hostile" player and do not have the temperament to get your exercise in this way. Instead of subjecting yourself to this dangerous kind of stress, get your exercise in a non-competitive endeavor such as jogging, swimming or jumping rope.

With any form of exercise, remember to always start your workout slowly and increase the intensity gradually. And when you stop, slow down gradually.

Gene McDougall

4. BLOOD TESTS

Throughout 1988 and 1989 I took part in a two year HEART DISEASE REVERSAL PROGRAM at Chicago's River City Medical Center, conducted by noted researcher, Dr. Michael Davidson, a truly amazing young man who is currently the President and CEO of the Chicago Center for Clinical Research as well as Director of Preventive Cardiology at Chicago's prestigious Rush-Presbyterian-St. Luke's Medical Center. It was while participating in his 1988-89 Heart Disease Reversal program that I started taking Lovistatin (more about that later) and learned about the critical blood level numbers to shoot for in order to reverse coronary artery disease **(cholesterol under 150, LDL under 100, VLDL under 30, total cholesterol/HDL ratio under 3.5, triglycerides under 150 and LDL/HDL ratio under 2.)**

To keep track of my progress, I get a Comprehensive Metabolic Panel blood test three times

28

a year. I suggest that you do the same. However, if and when certain new medications are introduced into your regimen, you may need more frequent blood tests for a while to more closely monitor their effect on your liver or kidney functions. For each blood test, a printout will be generated that should include everything on the following table (Table 1) and more. However, you may never get a copy of the complete printout unless you ask for it, so be sure to make it clear that you do want a copy for your records. You paid for it and it belongs to you.

To keep Table 1 from being too crowded, I tracked only the numbers for total cholesterol, HDL, LDL, VLDL, triglycerides, fasting blood sugar and glycohemoglobin, leaving out creatinine, bun/creatinine ratio, sodium, potassium, chloride, calcium, total protein, albumin, globulin, albumin/creatinine ratio, total bilirubin, alkaline phosphate and AST (SGOT). Just because I left these numbers out of the table does not mean they are not

Gene McDougall

important. I will briefly explain the significance of each of them later on in this chapter.

Table 1 displays the results of my blood tests from December of 1981 through December of 2000. Obviously, my weight and blood pressure were not part of the blood test printouts. I added them as benchmarks.

Table I - Blood counts

DATE	CHOL	HDL	LDL	VLDL	TG	FBS	GLYCO-HEMOG	WT	BLOOD PRESSURE
12/12/81					345	171			
4/22/84	213				258	182			
7/07/86						104		172	124/83
5/28/87	177	31	113		165	134		158	130/87
1/28/88	204	41	135		139	132	5.5	163	
3/25/88	182	40	132		52	124		159	
6/03/88	168	49	110	9	44	109		160	104/62
8/05/88	160	45	88	28	141	132		162	110/72
10/4/89	156	28	98	30	158	121	5.5	164	113/74
5/08/90	133	48	53	32	158	149	4.7	166	120/86
4/25/91	146	46	76	24	123	146	5.0	161	110/76
12/2/91	154	45	77	32	158	145	5.2	159	133/73
5/12/92	136	44	64	28	142	143	4.1	160	105/71
9/18/92	133	37	66	30	148	123	5.5	163	133/77
1/08/93	141	43	72	26	132	151	5.4	160	134/84
9/24/93	147	40	62	45	226	111	5.5	161	122/77
8/23/94	145	44	74	34	167	118	6.7	163	133/79
11/22/94	138	40	72	26	160	155	6.2	161	131/78
3/23/95	132	43	65	24	152	142	6.7	160	137/89
11/20/95	146	48	75	23	141	150	6.0	161	127/77
3/12/96	144	43	79	23	142	146	6.5	163	136/76
5/23/96	147	40	74	33	202	149	6.7	167	113/71
10/08/96	133	40	66	27	171	159	6.7	165	128/74
5/13/97	164	43	94	27	166	151	6.6	159	133/77
6/18/97	178	44	93	41	204	159	6.3	164	142/79
7/25/97	174	49	96	28	144	140	6.7	164	130/80
9/12/97	166	48	97	21	106	127	7.0	157	137/80
11/25/97	162	31	85	24	130	143	6.3	163	137/69
1/30/98	146	49	75	22	111	125	6.3	169	145/80
3/24/98	164	53	86	25	126	156	5.8	170	134/77
9/23/98	161	62	81	16	88	125	6.1	169	134/79
4/06/99	138	46	77	15	75	125	6.2	169	135/73
9/30/99	151	54	77	20	99	114	5.9	172	144/81
2/25/00	139	58	68	13	65	133	6.3	173	139/77
6/10/00	144	57	64	22	114	100	5.6	172	127/77
12/05/00	133	53	65	15	75	101	6.2	177	135/86

Gene McDougall

- **Total cholesterol:** Normal range is 140 to 200 mg. Keeping it under 150 for five years will reverse coronary artery disease. The average or normal range for cholesterol as well as all other categories in your blood test printout will change depending upon the most current medical thinking at the time, but the most recent "reference range" for each item will always appear on your printout and each item not within those parameters will be flagged.

- **HDL:** The "good" cholesterol which sweeps fat out of the arteries. Normal range for men is 29 mg to 67 mg - and for women, 35 mg to 86 mg. Something about the estrogen in the chemistry of women gives them some added protection. Regular exercise can raise HDL levels.

- **LDL:** "Bad" cholesterol - clogs the arteries. Normal is under 130, borderline is 130 to 160 and greater than 160 is high. Keep it under 100 to reverse clogging. Some labs do not include LDL in the Comprehensive Metabolic Panel, and if you request it you may find that you will be charged as much as $14 extra just because the figure was calculated in the doctor's office instead of the lab. Save your money. Do not ask for the LDL. You can easily make the calculation yourself from the numbers already included in your blood test printout. Just divide your triglycerides by five, add that number to your HDL and subtract the result from your total cholesterol. Using my 9/24/93 blood test as an example, my TG figure was 226. Dividing that by five gives us 45. Adding that 45 to my HDL (which was 40) gives us 85, and subtracting the 85 from my total cholesterol of 147 leaves 62 (my LDL). A little later on, I will tell you about some ratios that are important to you, why they are important, and how you can calculate them yourself using the numbers on your printout.

Gene McDougall

- **VLDL:** Another bad component of cholesterol. Keeping it under 30 can reverse atherosclerosis. You may have to calculate this one yourself also. Simply add the LDL and HDL numbers and subtract the result from your total cholesterol. Again using my 9/24/93 figures, add 40 and 62 and subtract the total (102) from 147. This gives you the VLDL figure of 45.

- **TG:** Triglycerides are neutral fat. Normal range is 50 mg to 200 mg. Keeping this count under 150 can reverse blockages. High TG levels inhibit the oxygen-carrying capacity of the blood. Exercise, proper diet and weight loss can lower TG.

- **FBS:** Fasting blood sugar (glucose): Normal is 65 to 125. Levels under 50 or over 150 should not be ignored.

- **GLYCOHEMOGLOBIN:** This shows the average glucose level over the previous three-month period. The normal range is between 3.9 and 6.3.

- **WEIGHT:** After my heart attack I brought my weight down about 15 pounds. It was not difficult. I will show you how I did it in the next chapter when I discuss nutrition. I am five feet 11 1/2 inches tall, so the weight I maintained for many years (160) was quite slim (skinny, actually) but healthy. I have gained some weight back lately, but I am currently addressing that issue and will soon reach my target of between 165 and 170.

- **BLOOD PRESSURE:** Normal is 120/80. If the first number (systolic) exceeds 140 or the second number (diastolic) exceeds 90, you have hypertension and steps to control it should be considered. Though you may have no symptoms, the long-term effects can be so destructive that undetected, untreated high blood pressure has come to be known as "the silent killer".

As mentioned earlier, the Comprehensive Metabolic Panel blood test yields much more information than I had room for on Table 1, so let me list some of the important numbers that were not on the table but will be on your printout:

- **BUN:** Urea nitrogen measures protein breakdown product in the blood that is removed by the kidney. Normal is 9 to 29. Higher levels signal possible kidney damage.

- **CREA:** Creatinine - the normal range is .8 to 1.5. A higher number is another sign of possible kidney damage.

- **BUN/CREA:** The BUN/Creatinine ratio is yet another index of kidney function. The average range is 6 to 27, with the optimum range being 6 to 20. The closer the numbers are to the low end of the scale, the healthier the kidney function.

- **URIC:** Uric acid - the normal range is 3.3 to 9.1. Eating less protein can lower this number. Obesity, diabetes or high blood pressure could raise it.

- **CA:** Calcium - normal range is 8.4 to 10.3.

- **PHOS:** Phosphate - normal range is 2.1 to 4.1.

- **LDH (or LD-L):** Lactate dehydrogenase. An enzyme secreted in the liver, heart muscle, brain, etc. Normal range is 115 to 260. Numbers out of this range could signal the need for further testing.

- **AST (SGOT):** Measures liver function. Normal is 1 to 45.

- **ALT (SGPT):** Another measure of liver function. Normal range is between 1 and 50.

- **ALP:** Alkaline phosphatose, another liver enzyme. Normal is 45 to 196.

- **GGT:** Gamma glut. transpeptidase is another liver enzyme. Normal is 8 to 62.

- **TBIL:** Total bilirubin. Normal range is .3 to 1.4. Numbers out of that range could signal liver damage.

- **ALB:** Albumin - normal range is 3.7 to 5.2.

- **A/G ratio:** This is the ratio between albumin and globulin. The normal range is 1.0 to 2.0. Numbers outside that range could indicate certain disease states.

- **TP:** Total protein. Normal range is 6.0 to 8.0.

- **MG:** Manganese. Normal is 1.8 to 2.6.

- **IRON:** Normal is 20 to 160.

- **NA:** Sodium. Normal is 133 to 145.

- **Potassium.** Normal is 3.4 to 5.1.

- **Chloride (salt).** Normal is 96 to 108.

- **CO2:** Carbon dioxide. Normal is 21 to 31.

Two ratios that are important to you but may not appear on your printout are:

- **Total cholesterol/HDL:** Arrived at by dividing total cholesterol by HDL. Strive to keep this number under 3.5. My 9/24/93 cholesterol of 147 divided by my HDL of 40 was 3.68 - just a little too high. An HDL of just two points higher (42) would have brought the ratio down to 3.5. The needed improvement in my HDL numbers did not occur until 1988 when I started taking Lovistatin.

- **LDL/HDL:** LDL divided by HDL. The magic number here is 2. Keep it under 2 and coronary artery disease can be reversed. Again, using my 9/24/93 blood test as an example, my LDL of 62 divided by my HDL of 40 resulted in an LDL/HDL ratio of 1.55, which was excellent.

5. NUTRITION

It is not possible to successfully combat atherosclerosis without paying close attention to diet. In my case, what I eat is even more important because of my diabetes. Fortunately, the same eating habits are helpful for both conditions.

The American Diabetes Association recommends plenty of fruits and vegetables, whole grains and other high fiber foods - and less fat and sugar. Everyone, diabetic or not, should follow these same general guidelines. More specifically, carbohydrate intake should be 55-60% of calories - concentrate on complex carbohydrates (starches) such as brown rice, pasta and whole grain breads, rather than simple carbohydrates (sugar) - protein should account for 15-20% of calories, fiber intake should be 30-40 grams a day, cholesterol under 300 mg, sodium under 3,000 mg and fat under 30% of calories (10% saturated, 10% polyunsaturated and 10% monunsaturated). Less fat

41

than this would be even better, especially if replaced by carbohydrates rather than protein. Avoid saturated fats as you would poison. They are more likely to cause health problems than cholesterol in the diet.

Although I love to chase tennis balls around for hours at a time, I am basically a lazy person. So when I was first introduced to the diabetic food exchange meal regimen, I was so overwhelmed and horrified that I decided to look for another way.

The most widely used method of controlling weight is simply counting calories. Just decide how many pounds you want to weigh, multiply that by 15 and consume that many calories per day. For instance, if you are - or want to be - 150 pounds, just eat 2250 calories (150 x 15) a day. If you have normal metabolism and already weigh 150, this will keep you there. If you do not weigh 150, this will eventually get you there. Of course, the more you exercise, the more calories you can eat and still achieve your goal.

I do remain aware of my calorie intake, but that is definitely not my main focus. Instead, I count the grams of fat consumed. I have found that it is not possible for me to gain weight if I eat no more than 50 grams of fat a day. And I make sure that most of that fat is not the saturated type. Monounsaturated is the least harmful, with polyunsaturated being the next best choice. I also avoid any product containing hydrogenated or partially hydrogenated fat. These are what is known an trans fats, which start out as mono or polyunsaturated, but for commercial purposes are chemically changed into fats which may be even more deleterious to your health than saturated (animal) fats.

Avoiding trans fats automatically eliminates most frozen dinners as well as a large percentage of packaged foods found in the local supermarkets. Also eliminated are most margarines, even the ones labeled "light".

Only 50 grams of fat per day may sound like a sacrifice to some people, but taste is an acquired thing

43

and I have gradually lost all interest in high fat foods such as steaks, hot dogs or hamburgers. Although red meat is out, I eat chicken and try to eat fish at least twice a week. I used to hate fish, but knowing something is good for you makes it more appealing, and I now enjoy many different types of cold-water fish.

I didn't have to acquire a taste for spaghetti. I've loved it all my life, so I enjoy some vermicelli at least once a week. There are lots of low fat soups around. My favorite is Healthy Choice. A can of one of these soups with some left over elbow macaroni thrown in makes a great lunch.

Want a healthy, filling, good-tasting breakfast you'll never get tired of? Try any one of the following cereals (I often mix them all together in one bowl), with a little soymilk and some fruit slices:

General Mills Fiber One

Lifestream Flax Plus

Veri-pure Puffed Kashi

Nature's Path Multi-Grain Oatbran Flakes
Kashi GoLean.

Although I seldom eat eggs, there are quite a few
excellent egg substitutes now on the market. I use
Fleischmann's refrigerated Egg Beaters. Often, for
breakfast or lunch, I will pour a 3.4 ounce container in
a bowl that has been lightly sprayed with Olive Oil
PAM, and then microwave it for just under 3 minutes.
This is good with toast or on top of a small (3.5 ounce)
President's Choice Splendido Original Italian Bread
Shell which has been heated in the microwave 40
seconds. I buy these at my local Jewel store, but many
other supermarket chains have a comparable product.
Safeway's, for instance, is Select Verdi Original Italian
Style Flatbread.

Most bread is fattening and unhealthy. If it says
"enriched," that is your tip-off that all the good stuff
has been taken out and bad stuff such as preservatives
have been added. But there is one brand of bread that

is so healthy and delicious that I often have a slice for dessert or as a snack. The bread, bagels and muffins made by Natural Ovens of Manitowoc Wisconsin are actually that good. Not only that, but they are healthy and nutritious.

Their Multi-Grain Bread and Sunny Millet Whole Grain Bread and are two of my favorites. They also have many other tasty breads, such as 100% Whole Grain. They are all so good that they really need no spread at all, but for variety I will sometimes toast a slice and spread on some fat-free Philadelphia cream cheese or sugar free jelly. They also have delicious bagels, cookies and buns. Try them all. I have one of their carrot muffins just about every day.

I talked with Natural Ovens owner Paul Stitt recently about his products, and when I explained the purpose of my book, he told me about one of his newest products which he felt would be helpful in keeping my arteries open and my cardiovascular system healthy. It's called UltraOmega Balance, the

46

Ultimate Energy Mix with 2000 mg if Omega-3 and 525 ORAC units of antioxidants! It's a one-pound box of powder with ground flaxseed, extracts of sorghum and grape seed containing high levels of polyphenols, soy extract and inulin.

A tablespoon can be mixed with juice, water, or a combination of the two. So, since I had already been drinking a glass of water and orange juice with a spoonful of Metamucil every noon, I have simply added a tablespoon of UltraOmega to my daily "cocktail."

Natural Ovens of Manitowoc products are not nationally distributed, but they are so good for you and so delicious that you may want to order some directly from their bakery if you do not live in Wisconsin, Minneapolis or Chicago where their line is currently available in stores. More about that, but first a few words about Paul Stitt.

He earned his master's degree in biochemistry at the University of Wisconsin, and as a recognized expert in the field of health and nutrition, he has made promoting good health his mission in life. Although he had been running a multi-million dollar business for years, Mr. Stitt was taking only an average working man's salary for himself. Finally, the Internal Revenue Service put a stop to it. Feeling that they were not collecting their fair share of taxes, the IRS decided he was underpaid and that changes would have to be made, so his salary was increased. He then set up a system whereby half the company's profits would go to his employees and the other half to the company's growth, putting an end to his long-standing policy of not expanding his market beyond Wisconsin, Chicago and Minneapolis. As a result, Natural Ovens is set to break ground for a new plant in Valparaiso, Indiana in the spring of 2001 and expects to be baking bread there by the spring of 2002. This will expand their distribution area to include not only the original markets of Wisconsin, Chicago and Minneapolis, but also the additional markets of St. Louis, Michigan, Ohio and Indiana.

Unfortunately, even with this expansion, Natural Ovens products will not be available in retail outlets nationally. But even if you do not live within their marketing area, you can order products from their bakery by calling them at 1-800-772-0730 or 1-800-558-3535. If you have a computer, you can order or obtain information by logging on to their website "naturalovens.com." This site is currently being set up so should it be operational by the time this book is published.

Now on to the business of setting up and tracking a nutritional plan of your own. The next few pages will show you how. After you get used to it, keeping track of your consumption of fat grams, carbohydrates and so forth is not that hard. Most commercial products have these counts listed on the package. You just have to be aware that these numbers refer not to the contents of the entire package, but to "serving sizes" which are often unrealistically small - so a little math is required. There are no numbers provided for such things as fruit, vegetables and meat - but we don't want to eat red meat anyhow, do we? At any rate, the figures you will need for all those things can be found in books such as "The Complete Book of Food Counts" by Corinne T. Netzer. For each food item, she shows the number of calories as well as the grams of protein, carbohydrates, fat, cholesterol, sodium and fiber.

Get her book or one like it and then track your calorie, protein, carbohydrate, cholesterol, sodium and fiber intake for a few days. I have done that on the following table (Table 2), posting the food I ate on a day picked at random. As it turned out, I did not eat the most healthy or balanced diet on that particular day (no fruits or vegetables at all), and since this was years ago, some of the products listed might no longer even exist, but let's use that table anyhow. All my numbers were on target or better except for sodium (salt). It is best to keep that number lower than I did that day because, in addition to possibly causing high blood pressure, high sodium intake increases hunger. Table 3 is a blank version of Table 2. Make copies of it and use it to track your own consumption of calories, protein, carbohydrate, cholesterol, sodium and fiber. You may be surprised when you discover how healthy or unhealthy your eating habits really are.

Notice that there is a place on Table 3 where you can multiply the grams of protein and carbohydrates by four and the grams of fat by nine. That is because one gram of protein or carbohydrates will produce four calories while one gram of fat produces nine. Once you start posting all the numbers on the packages you buy, you will begin to realize that the sum of the parts (protein, carbohydrates and fat), after being multiplied by four, four and nine respectively, will seldom equal the total calories printed on the package. Since the manufacturers' figures are sometimes overstated and sometimes understated, there doesn't seem to be a conspiracy. Anyhow, to make things come out right, you will see an "S.O.P" entry on the table. That stands for "sum of the parts"- which means I have added the protein, carbohydrate and fat calories together to arrive at the correct total figure of 2331.2. Obviously, this does not agree with the 2295 derived from totaling the column for calories listed on the packages. The 2331.2 figure (sum of the parts) is therefore the one I used to figure percentages. Had I not done so, the sum of the parts would have been 102% of the total. If you do not mind the figures being off a few points, you needn't go through all that. Just use the manufacturers' figures and you will be close.

Singles tennis burns off about 420 calories an hour, and since I played an hour and a half of singles tennis that day, we subtract 630 calories from my intake of 2331. This puts my net intake at 1701 calories for the day, which was not enough to maintain my weight - yet I was munching all day long. To find out how many calories various activities will burn off, just find one of the many such lists which periodically appear in health magazines, books and newspapers. If you have seen a few of these lists, you will have noticed that they are not consistent. This is because there are so many variables. Your weight, how eagerly you pursue the activity and your individual metabolism are just a few of the many reasons why any such figures can only be approximate.

However, as I have said, calorie counting is not the way I have chosen to control my nutritional intake. Not only do the manufacturers' own packages contain inconsistencies, but, as Paul Stitt points out in his book, "Why Calories Don't Count", each of us has his or her own basal metabolism rate - the minimum energy we must expend in order to live. The more active we are, the more our energy needs increase, but by how much? That depends on our age, health, body weight and generic inheritance. According to Mr. Stitt, the body hungers not just for carbohydrates, protein and fat, but for a full complement of the vitamins, minerals and other nutrients needed for

53

optimal health. Only when those needs have been met will hunger be abated. He feels that eating natural rather than processed foods is important if this is to be achieved, and I agree.

The importance of fiber deserves a special mention here. Your fiber intake plays a crucial role in controlling your digestive system, and an efficiently functioning digestive system is essential for good health. About 30 grams of fiber a day is generally a good target to shoot for, but it may not be right for everyone. Your bowel habits will tell you what is right for you. If you are passing marble-like stools, you need more fiber. If you are having bowel movements several times a day and they are loose, you are probably consuming too much fiber. If your stools are firm, easily passed and have the circumference of a quarter, you're right on target. I don't know about you, but this is starting to bum me out. Let's move on.

TABLE 2 - Calorie chart

Item	Calories	Protein grams	Carbo grams	Fat grams	Chol mg	Sodium mg	Fiber grams
BREAKFAST							
Egg Beaters	*50*	*10*	*2*	*0*	*0*	*160*	*0*
Pres Choice Splendido 3.5 oz	*270*	*10*	*48*	*3*	*0*	*470*	*0*
Nat. Ovens Cranberry Muffin	*195*	*6*	*34*	*5*	*0*	*100*	*4*
Orange Juice 6 oz	*76*	*1*	*18*	*.2*	*0*	*2*	*0*
LUNCH							
Veggie Burger	*110*	*5*	*19*	*3*	*0*	*370*	*0*
Bun	*130*	*4*	*21*	*3*	*0*	*260*	*0*
Healthy Choice Soup	*120*	*3*	*23*	*1*	*0*	*540*	*0*
DINNER							
Vermicelli 6 oz	*630*	*21*	*126*	*2*	*0*	*0*	*0*
Gianotti Pasta Sauce 4 oz	*55*	*2*	*7*	*0*	*0*	*390*	*1*
Nat.Oven Nutty Bread 6 slices	*240*	*12*	*48*	*4*	*0*	*560*	*12*
SNACKS							
Cape Cod Popcorn 3.5 oz	*210*	*7*	*28*	*10*	*0*	*333*	*14*
Joseph's cookies (3)	*94*	*2.7*	*12*	*3.9*	*0*	*12*	*1.2*
Nat.Oven Glorious Bread 2 sl	*90*	*6*	*22*	*.5*	*0*	*80*	*6*
Kraft Fat Free Phil C Ch 1 oz	*25*	*4*	*1*	*0*	*5*	*170*	*0*
TOTALS	*2295*	*93.7*	*409*	*35.6*	*5*	*3447*	*38.2*
MULTIPLIERS	*S. O. P.*	*x 4*	*x 4*	*x 9*			
CALORIES	*2331.2*	*374.8*	*1636*	*320.4*		*3447*	*38.2*
TARGET (< = less than)	*2400*	**15-20%**	**55-60%**	**< 30%**	**< 300**	**< 3000**	**30-40**
ACTUAL	*2331.2*	*16%*	*70%*	*14%*	*5*	*3447*	*38.2*

Gene McDougall

TABLE 3 - Calorie chart

Item	Calories	Protein grams	Carbo grams	Fat grams	Chol mg	Sodium mg	Fiber grams
TOTALS							
MULTIPLIERS	*S. O. P.*	*x 4*	*x 4*	*x 9*			
CALORIES							
TARGET (< = less than)		15-20%	55-60%	< 30%	< 300	< 3000	30-40
ACTUAL							

6. PILLS

All my life I have been told that if I eat properly I do not need vitamin supplements. Hogwash! Taking certain vitamins far in access of the RDA (Recommended Daily Allowance) can work miracles. This is not to say that if a little is good, huge amounts are always better. Going overboard on some vitamins or minerals could be toxic.

Pills of any kind are not something you should pop into your mouth without knowing what they can do for you or to you. Case in point - aspirin. Many people with atherosclerosis, and many doctors as well, do not realize that taking a regular 325 mg aspirin every day to reduce cardiac risk could be overkill and defeat the purpose. Here's why. While a 100 mg dose of aspirin will inhibit the clumping together of platelets that can cause blood clotting, larger doses tend to decrease the production of prostacyclin, which is an anti-clotting agent. Therefore, a regular aspirin every other day, or

57

a baby aspirin every day would be the proper amount to protect against blood clots.

Another thing about aspirin - too much of it could damage the stomach and cause bleeding. That's why I take Ecotrin instead of aspirin. Ecotrin is basically nothing more than aspirin with an enteric coating added to protect the stomach lining.

For more than a decade, I have kept a record of every event I felt might affect my health. When matched against my blood tests over those years, some interesting cause-and-effect relationships emerge. The most obvious of these concerns Lopid, which I began using in March of 1988 with spectacular results. My triglycerides immediately dropped to one-third of their previous levels and stayed there until I replaced Lopid with Lovistatin three months later:

Table 4 - Lopid

Date	Changes in medication	Triglycerides	SGOT (AST)
1/28/88		139	
3/05/88	Began Lopid 300 mg		
3/25/88		42	
6/03/88		44	45
6/04/88	Switched from Lopid to Lovistatin		
8/05/88		135	24

As you can see, the figure for SGOT (AST), a liver enzyme, was 45 in June, higher than my previous readings had always been, and outside the 10 to 42 range which was considered normal at that time. (The parameters have since been broadened and are now 1 to 45.) Anyhow, after switching to Lovistatin, my SGOT (AST) reading went right back down to normal where it has remained ever since.

Clofibrate, which is chemically similar to Lopid, has caused liver cancer in rats. This does not mean it will do the same thing to humans, but my liver enzymes did shoot up dramatically so it did not seem

Gene McDougall

prudent for me to stick with Lopid, especially since its long term use can also cause gallstones.

Another interesting finding produced by my journal concerned kidney stones and magnesium. The following table tells the story:

Table 5 - Magnesium

Date	Changes in medication	Event
1/18/87		Lithotripsy (shock wave kidney stone removal)
3/25/88	Began magnesium 30 mg	
1/27/91		Passed stone
8/01/91	Increased magnesium to 330 mg	
10/11/91		Passed stone
6/09/92		Passed stone
9/27/92	Increased magnesium to 630 mg	
11/10/93	Decreased magnesium to 530 mg	

I have had no more kidney stones since increasing my magnesium intake to 630 mg daily in September of 1992. The only reason I decreased the amount from 630 to 530 mg in November of 1993 was because

Walgreens discontinued their 300 mg tablets in favor of 250 mg tablets at that time. (In case you were wondering about that extra 30 mg, I was taking a multivitamin during that period that contained 30 mg of magnesium. Thanks for asking.)

Charting the proper course has not always been easy. Not everything in print can be blindly accepted. There are snake oil salesmen all over the place and my biggest challenge was to separate the good guys from the bad guys. This also applies to doctors. They range all the way from magnificent to downright dangerous. During the period when I was working on this project, I developed a rather alarming rash on my left temple. My internist sent my to an allergist who correctly diagnosed the rash as shingles, but failed to prescribe the proper treatment. After a week of increasingly painful headaches, I finally did what I should have done much earlier - I researched the disease, beginning with a fine book I keep in my home, "The Best Treatment" by Dr. Isadore Rosenfeld. (Buy it!) Now realizing that I had not been receiving the right treatment, I called my internist. As soon as I told him I had shingles, he prescribed exactly what Dr. Rosenfeld had prescribed - Zovirax 800 mg, 5 or 6 times a day for 10 days. I was lucky. Even though the treatment was started late, I recovered completely in a couple of weeks.

The allergist in question certainly represents one kind of doctor to avoid. Also stay away from any doctor who is too busy or uninterested in you as a person to answer your questions satisfactorily. You have every right to know the complete details of your medical condition as well as the full particulars regarding each medication or procedure which could be involved in your treatment. To be effective, you and your doctor should both consider yourselves partners in your health care. If he is unwilling to sit down and discuss all your questions with you, fire him on the spot. Or, if confrontation makes you uncomfortable, you can fire him by just never going back. It is important for you to have confidence in your doctor because this automatically provides you with an additional weapon in your battle to get well. It is called the placebo effect. The proper mental attitude, the belief that you are on the right track and will prevail, has been proven time and time again to be a powerful influence in successfully overcoming seemingly hopeless medical problems. The brain releases natural healing chemicals throughout the body all the time, but this function is definitely enhanced when you send the right signals. Do that by having an upbeat, resolute, confident attitude, combined with a tenacious determination to succeed.

A few words of explanation about my journal (Table 6) are in order:

3/4/92

I switched from Cardizem SR to Cardizem CD primarily for the convenience of being able to take just

Gene McDougall

one capsule a day instead of two, since the CD version is longer lasting.

10/2/92

I began taking Coenzyme Q10 even though the jury was still out on whether there is any value in doing so. Still, since it was an anti-oxidant and could do no harm except to the wallet, I chose to include it in my vitamin program. Years later, the jury finally did come in. It was decided that there was no proven benefit associated with the product (so I quit taking it when my supply ran out on December 31, 2000).

2/10/93

I quit taking lecithin after reading that commercial lecithin supplements are of no value in lowering cholesterol levels.

11/7/92

At a diabetes seminar I attended in November of 1992, I learned that Glucotrol should be taken 1/2 hour before meals to keep the blood sugar level from bouncing around. I did that for about a year, decided it made no difference in the control of my blood sugar, and then went back to the more convenient method of taking Glucotrol with my other pills at mealtime. Later, I switched from Glucotrol to Glucophage - which should be taken <u>with</u> (rather than before) meals. Still later, I switched to Rezulin until it was taken off the market because it was causing fatal liver damage to some people. So I then switched to another drug in the same family, Actos, which I take in conjunction with glyburide, another diabetes drug. Obviously, it is important to stay alert to the rapid advances in the medical field so that you will always be getting the best treatment currently available.

Gene McDougall

10/07/96

The May 2, 1996 New England Journal of Medicine reported that a recently concluded 12-year study found that taking beta carotene supplements "produced neither benefit nor harm" for over 22,000 male physicians (age 40 to 84). It therefore seemed reasonable to assume that the improvement found in the blood flow to my heart was due to the other factors listed rather than the beta carotene I started taking in 1992 (see Table 8) - so I discontinued it. I have since resumed taking it, then reduced and increased the dosage depending on the latest published studies, (i.e.; it is bad for ex-smokers, good for the lining of the intestines, etc.) Currently I am taking 5,000 IU a day as part of a multi-vitamin pill.

Well, you get the idea. No need for me to continue describing each and every medication change in I made over the years. These changes were usually made because of all the new and better drugs coming into the

66

marketplace as well as new studies adding to our knowledge of herbs, vitamins and minerals. Nor will I burden you with the dozens of entries in my journal that have no direct bearing on my fight against atherosclerosis. Most of those entries have been deleted from the tables. The following is a case in point

In March of 2000, I began a daily early morning stretching ritual to help my Achilles tendons, knees, hamstrings and back. While still on my back in bed, I bring one knee up to touch my nose (this stretches the knees and back), and while still in that position, I pull my toes towards my face (stretching my Achilles tendon). I then stick my leg straight up toward ceiling as far as possible (to stretch the hamstring). I repeat the same stretches with the other leg. About five minutes of this is all it takes. My journal indicates that all the foot, heel, Achilles tendon and back problems that used to be so common have been almost completely eliminated since a began those stretches. You will not see all those dozens of postings in my journal, because, in order to spare you many, many pages of documentation, I deleted most of the entries describing my aches and pains. Also, you will be pleased to know I deleted the dozen or so entries pertaining to the allergist from hell whom I discussed earlier. Did I mention that his receptionist was a chain smoker who had an ashtray full of butts on the sign-in counter?

I'm sure you would not have wanted to plow through the unabridged version of my journal, but I'm glad I had all those postings available for my own review. I strongly urge you to keep a journal of your own to match against your blood tests. Your doctor cannot be expected to do this for you, yet you can see that keeping good records can result in the discovery of some valuable cause-and-effect relationships.

Here's another example to further illustrate my point:

On January 26 of 2001, an interesting story appeared on the evening news. A three-year study had shown that taking 1,500 mg of Glucosamine daily had stopped osteoarthritis in its tracks, preventing any further knee cartilage deterioration during that period.

In the past, I had taken Glucosamine for a while, but had discontinued it because at that time there had been no proof that it was effective against osteoarthritis, and there was some concern about whether it raised blood sugar levels. But now, in light of this latest news, my interest in Glucosamine was rekindled.

I looked back through my journal and found that from January 13 of 1998 through February 13 of 2000 I had been taking two Chondroitin Complex tablets daily, each tablet containing 400 mg of Glucosamine.

I then looked back over my blood test table to see what my glychohemoglobin counts were for the periods before, during and after my taking

Glucosamine. Table 5a shows that the Glucosamine made no significant difference in my blood sugar.

Table 5a - Glucosamine

Action	Date	Glycho-hemoglobin	Average
	5/13/97	6.6	
	6/15/97	6.3	
	7/25/97	6.7	6.58
	9/12/97	7.0	
	11/25/97	6.3	
Began 800 Glucosamine daily	1/13/98		
	1/30/98	6.3	
	3/24/98	5.8	
	9/23/98	6.1	6.06
	4/06/98	6.2	
	9/30/99	5.9	
Quit Glucosamine	2/10/00		
	2/25/00	6.3	
	6/10/00	5.6	6.03
	12/05/00	6.2	

But wait. The plot thickens. During this same period, I also made several changes in my diabetes medications. In September of 1997, my doctor decided that we should keep tighter control of my diabetes, so he added 2.5 mg of glyburide to the 600 mg of Rezulin

I was already taking. Glyburide is a second-generation sulfonylurea which stimulates the pancreas to secrete more insulin. Rezulin is a thiazolidlinedione which reduces cellular resistance to insulin. Combining these two approaches worked very well in controlling my diabetes, but in May of 2000, the FDA took Rezulin off the market because the mortality rate due to liver damage had became too great. Since Rezulin had worked well for me, and my blood tests showed no adverse effects on my liver, I switched to another thiazolidlinedione, Actos.

All these changes in my diabetes medication muddied the water, turning Table 5a into the more complex Table 5b. Still, my glychohemoglobin had remained within an acceptable range all through the period when these changes were made, so what did all this mean? Simply that Glucosamine had little or no effect on my blood sugar during that time, and that any changes that might occur in the future could be controlled by just fine-tuning my diabetic medication.

Gene McDougall

Therefore, I plan to add Glucosamine to my daily supplements.

Table 5b - Glucosamine, Rezulin, glyburide, Actos

Action	Date	Glycho-hemoglobin	Average
	5/13/97	6.6	
	6/15/97	6.3	
	7/25/97	6.7	6.58
Rezulin from 400 mg to 600 mg	8/25/97		
	9/12/97	7.0	
Add glyburide 2.5 mg	9/25/97		
	11/25/97	6.3	
Began 800 Glucosamine daily	1/13/98		
	1/30/98	6.3	
	3/24/98	5.8	
	9/23/98	6.1	6.06
Rezulin from 600 mg to 400 mg	11/08/98		
Rezulin from 400 mg to 200 mg	11/23/98		
	4/06/98	6.2	
Rezulin from 200 mg to 400 mg	1/02/99		
Rezulin from 400 mg to 600 mg	1/09/99		
glyburide from 2.5 mg to 5 mg	3/11/99		
	9/30/99	5.9	
Quit Glucosamine	2/10/00		
	2/25/00	6.3	
Quit Rezulin	5/11/00		6.03
Began Actos 30 mg	5/18/00		
	6/10/00	5.6	
	12/05/00	6.2	

TABLE 6 - MY JOURNAL

Code	Date	Item **** = Thallium stress test results
	1981	Good boss retired, replaced by bad one
	1981	Brother died
	1982	Mother died
MA	1984	Marital problems surfaced
	4/02/86	Started low fat diet
GL	6/05/86	Started Glucotrol 5 mg
	6/22/86	Heart attack
	7/31/86	Bypass surgery
F P EC	9/30/86	Started 8 fish oil, 1 Persantine and 1 Ecotrin 325 mg daily
F	1/12/87	Stopped fish oil
	1/18/87	Lithotripsy (shock wave kidney stone removal)
	3/09/87	Retired
LO	3/05/88	Started Lopid 300 mg
V	3/25/88	Started vitamins and minerals
LO L	6/04/88	Started Lovistatin 20 mg, quit Lopid
CO	10/16/88	Started Colestid (2 packages daily)
CO	8/28/89	Quit Colestid, doubled C to 1810
L	11/23/89	Doubled Lovistatin to 40 mg
****	2/08/90	40% blood flow at peak exercise
	2/12/90	Put Gerne to sleep
	2/27/90	Cortisone shot for torn right rotator cuff
CA	3/15/90	Started Cardizem SR 180 mg (90x2)
GL	6/15/90	Increased Glucotrol from 5 mg to 10 mg
P EC	7/23/90	Quit Persantine, decreased Ecotrin 325 mg to 3xweekly
MA	10/10/90	Marital problem resolved (separated)

	1/27/91	Passed kidney stone
****	2/20/91	60% blood flow at peak exercise (that's better)
CA	2/22/91	Increased Cardizem SR to 240 mg (120x2)
	4/29/91	Bursitis in right knee (also happened a year or so ago) Knee brace and Naprosyn (4 daily) cured it in 10 days
Mg	8/01/91	Increased Magnesium from 30 mg to 330 mg
CR	9/08/91	Started chromium 200 mg
SR B	9/20/91	Started AARP Sr and AARP B Complex
	10/11/91	Passed kidney stone
M	11/22/91	Started Metamucil (psyllium) 1 tsp daily
Beta	1/10/91	Started 25,000 IU beta carotene
C	1/15/91	Reduced vitamin C to 810 mg
	6/27/91	Passed kidney stone
	10/11/91	Passed kidney stone at NW Community Hospital at 8:30 AM, just 30 minutes before my Urinoscopy would have begun
****	3/03/92	60% blood flow to the heart at peak exercise (no change)
CA	3/04/92	Switched from Cardizem SR to Cardizem CD (300 mg)
L Z	3/04/92	Switched from Lovistatin to Zocor 20 mg (10x2)
	6/09/92	Passed kidney stone
CR	6/28/92	Doubled chromium to 400 mg (200x2)
N	8/01/92	Increased niacin from 41 to 116 mg

C N	9/27/92	Decreased C from 820 to 610 and niacin from 116 to 66 mg
Mg B	9/27/92	Increased Magnesium from 330 to 630 and B12 from 13 to 53 mg
CR	9/27/92	Switched from chromium to chromium picolinate
Q LE	10/02/92	Started CoQ-10 (60 mg) and lethicin (2400 mg)
HYD	10/20/92	Quit hydrogenated oils (in most processed foods)
GL	11/07/92	Started taking Glucotrol ½ hour before meals
****	12/22/92	90% blood flow at peak exercise (much better)
	1/25/93	Blurred vision and dizziness while playing tennis today. Probably because of my diabetes. Will drink diluted orange juice or have a lifesaver as needed while playing in the future.
LE	2/10/93	Quit Lethicin
	3/19/93	Orange juice did the trick. No more problems.
	5/31/93	Quit peanut butter
GL	10/17/93	Resumed taking Glucotrol WITH meals
Mg	11/10/93	Decreased magnesium from 630 to 530 mg
C	11/11/93	Increased C from 610 to 1610
C E	1/18/94	C from 1610 to 1360. E from 1065 to 815
LY	1/29/94	Began Lysine 1000 mg
E	3/15/94	Increased E from 815 to 1015

C	3/22/94	1000 mg of C switched to Ester-C
CR	4/15/94	Switched from 400 mcg chromium picolinate to 200 mcg chromium picolinate and 200 mcg chromium GTF
C	10/05/94	C from 1360 to 2360 mg (including 2000 Ester-C)
GL	10/30/94	Glucotrol from 10 mg to 5 mg (2.5 x 2)
GL	11/12/94	Switched from Glucotrol to Glucotrol XL (5 mg)
GL	8/09/95	Switched from Glucotrol XL to Glucophage (500 mg x 2)
GL	8/31/95	Switched from Glucophage to Glucotrol XL (5 mg x 2)
CA	4/05/96	Cardizem CD from 300 mg to 180 mg
COZ	4/05/96	Began Cozaar 50 mg x 1
C	4/24/96	Decreased C from 2360 to 1360 (over 1000 could increase oxalate which can cause kidney stones)
	5/02/96	Resumed moderate intake of peanut butter (natural source of vit. E)
GL	7/09/96	Quit Glucotrol XL 5 mg x2, started Glucophage 500 mg x1 (Davidson)
Beta	10/07/96	Quit 25,000 IU beta carotene
CA	12/16/96	Quit Cardizem CD
LY	4/18/97	Quit Lysine (bad for diabetics)
CR	4/20/97	Quit Chromium GTF 200 mg. Continue 200 mg Chromium Picolinate
E	4/20/97	E reduced from 1015 to 830 mg
C	4/20/97	C reduced from 1360 to 590 mg
B12	5/10/97	B-12 from 53 to 9 mcg
E liq	5/11/97	Started E liquid in nostril (good results)
Lip Rez	5/23/97	Lipitor 10 mg replacing Zocor 20 mg Rezulin 200 mg reducing Glucophage

Z GL		from 1000 to 500 mg
Lip Rez GL	6/25/97	Rezulin from 200 to 400 mg Quit Glucophage 500 mg Lipitor from 10 to 20 mg
SJW	7/18/97	Started St. John's Wort as needed for depression
Inf	7/24/97	Began Inflam-X for knee pain (as advised by Carol, my neuromuscular therapist))
Rez GL	7/25/97	Rezulin from 400 to 200 mg Glucophage (metformin)500 mg started
Inf	7/31/97	Quit Inflam-X
Meta	7/31/97	Quit Metamucil
Rez	8/03/97	Rezulin doubled to 400 mg
Dura	8/04/97	Began 7 days of Duract for knee pain, even tho no pain exists (Lopez)
Dura	8/11/97	Quit Duract 25 mg x 2 (considered harmful to liver?)
Ibu	8/13/97	Quit regular long-term use of Ibuprofen which I started 7/30/97
Glu Rez	8/25/97	Stopped Glucophage and increased Rezulin from 400 to 600 mg
StJ	8/27/97	Started intermittent use of St. John's Wort 2 X daily (relaxant)
E	9/14/97	Reduced E from 830 to 430
Asa	9/18/97	Began Asacol 400 mg 2x daily for colitis - NSAI (non-steroidal anti-inflammatory) for colon (colitis)
Gly	9/25/97	Began glyburide 2.5 mg (1 a day) for tighter diabetes control.

Beta	10/15/97	Increased beta carotene from 5,000 to 25,000 IU - important in maintaining strong epithelium (the lining of the intestines)
B-6	10/15/97	Increased B-6 from 3 mg to 103 mg – to guard against kidney stones
Chon	10/15/97	Began Chondroitin Sulfate 250 mg x 2 = 500 mg daily
B12	10/26/97	B-12 increased from 9 to 59 mcg to lower homocystine & protect heart
Gink	12/7/97	Began Ginkgo Biloba 40 mg x 2 = 80 mg
St.Jo	12/7/97	Began St. John's Wort 300 mg x 2 = 600 mg
Evol	1/03/98	Began Evolve once daily (contains 25 mg tocotrienol)
C	1/03/98	Dropped Ester C 500 mg
Chon Cpx	1/13/98	Replaced Chondroitin Sulfate with Chondroitin Complex (x2) (Contains: Chondroitin 500 mg, Glucosamine 400 mg & C 167 mg)
St Jo	2/09/98	Decreased St Johns Wort from 600 to 300 mg
CR	3/15/98	Added chromium GTF 200 mg
Chon	3/20/98	Added chondroitin sulfate 250 mg (lunch)
Calc	4/10/98	Began calcium citrate 950 (200) mg x 2 = 400 mg
Lipo	4/25/98	Began Alpha Lipoic Acid 30 mg
Chon	6/01/98	Quit extra (lunchtime) chondroitin sulfate 250 mg
C	6/10/98	Resumed 500 mg Ester-C, bringing daily total from 423 to 923 mg
Gink	6/14/98	Reduced Ginkgo from 240 to 120 mg

Trin	6/25/98	Began Natren Healthy Trinity (probiotics) one a day - with food but away from other pills - to create better balance of bacteria in colon
Q	7/15/98	Switched from CoQ10 **caps** (**30**mg x 2) to CoQ10 **GEL** (**15**mg x 2)
Gink	10/8/98	Quit Ginkgo
Aloe	1028/98	Started Aloe Juice 1 ½ oz daily for colon and arthritis
St.Jo	10/28/98	Quit St.John's Wort – **could** adversely effect sexual performance
Rez	11/08/98	Rezulin from 600 to 400 mg
Rez	11/23/98	Rezulin from 400 to 200 mg
Rez	1/02/99	Rezulin from 200 to 400
Rez	1/09/99	Rezulin from 400 to 600
Paxil	2/03/99	Began PAXIL 20 mg one per day for depression
Lora	2/06/99	Began Lorazepam .5 mg twice daily for anxiety
Paxil	2/12/99	Began PAXIL
Lora	2/14/99	Quit Lorazepam (affects coordination)
Paxil	2/22/99	Quit PAXIL – blocks orgasms
Glyb	3/11/99	Doubled glyburide from 2.5 to 5 mg
Meta	3/11/99	Quit Metamucil
Chro	3/23/99	Quit Chromium Picolinate
Beta	3/25/99	Beta Carotine from 25k to 15k
SAM	4/02/99	Started SAM-e 100 mg x 2 (200 mg)
SAM	6/28/99	Increased SAM-e from 200 mg to 400 mg
B-12	7/28/99	B-12 from 59 mcg to 1009 mcg (to facilitate SAM-e effectiveness)
SAM	7/30/99	Increased SAM-e from 400 to 600 mg
Folat	8/04/99	Increased folate from 400 to 800 mcg (to help SAM-e)
Chro	9/10/99	Quit Chromium GTF

C	9/16/99	Vitamin C from 1423 mg to 923 mg
Arth	11/8/99	Started 15 days of Arthotic (for knees)
Chon	11/19/99	Quit Chondroitin Complex
Chon	12/04/99	Resumed Chondroitin Complex
	12/05/99	After tennis Friday, knees VERY painful all weekend.
Chon	12/07/99	MRI right knee- Increased chondroitin glucosomine from 2 to 3x daily
	12/26/99	Dr. Palella took 28 x-rays of knees, feet and hip
Synv	2/02/00	Palella drained both knees and injected SYNVISC. Injections scheduled twice more for a total of three injections. Should last about a year. Very painful shots, but wonderful results right away
Met	2/05/00	Resumed Metamucil
Chon	2/10/00	Quit Chondroiten Complex (Glucosamine raises blood suger)
Beta	2/25/00	Quit Beta Carotine, except for the 5,000 IU in Theravim-m (saw story in paper that it is bad for ex-smokers)
Trin	4/11/00	Quit Healthy Trinity
Lipo	4/23/00	Increased Alpha Lipoic Acid from 30 to 60 mg
Rez	5/11/00	Quit Rezulin 600 mg
Acto s	5/18/00	Started Actos 30 mg x 1
T#4	5/23/00	Started Tylenol #4 for neck cramp (for 4 days)
Chro	12/22/00	Started Chromium Picolinate 200mcgx2 for weight control

Gene McDougall

CoQ	12/31/00	Quit CoQ10
Ultra	1/17/01	Started UltraOmega 1 tablespoon daily
Synv SAM	2/02/01	One year since Synvisc shots and knees are still good. Cutting tennis down to only three times a week, stretching and taking 600 mg of SAM-e daily may also be helping

The first part of the next table (Table 7) consists primarily of the vitamins and. minerals I am currently taking. The last six lines of the table are prescription drugs; (1) Claritin, an antihistamine which I take in season for protection against ragweed and related allergies, (2) Asacol, which I take to control colitis and diverticulosis, (3) Cozaar, an angiotensin blocking agent (A-II receptor blocker) that lowers blood pressure by inhibiting the narrowing of blood vessel, and also improves insulin sensitivity, (4).glyburide, an oral sulfonylurea agent used to control diabetes, (5) Lipitor, an oral HMG-CoA reductase inhibitor, which lowers the total cholesterol, LDL (bad) cholesterol and tryglycerides while increasing the amount of HDL

82

(good) cholesterol in the blood and (6) Actos, an antihyperglycemic agent that reduces the amount of sugar produced by the liver. It also helps the body respond better to insulin. In short, it helps control blood sugar levels.

Table 7 - Vitamins/medications

1 gm = 1,000 mg 1 mg = 1,000 mcg	Individual Pills	Primary purpose	PuritanPride theravim-m	Daily Totals	OPTIMAL
Time of day to be taken →	as stated		dinner		
Alpha Lipoic Acid 30 mg	Bkfst Dinner	Heart and diabetes		60 mg	37-600 mg
Beta carotene	Dinner	Colon & heart artery lining	5,000 IU	5,000 IU	
B-1 (thiamin)			3 mg	3 mg	1.5 -10 mg
B-2 (Riboflavin)			3.4 mg	3.4 mg	1.7 - 10 mg
B-3 (niacin)			20 mg	20 mg	20- 200 mg
B-5 (pantothenate)			10 mg	10 mg	10 - 50 mg
B-6 (pyridoxine) 100 mg	Dinner	Colitis and kidney stones	3 mg	103 mg	20 mg
B-12 - 1000 mcg Sustained Release	Bkfst	Heart + assist to SAMe	9 mcg	1009 mcg	60 mcg
Folic Acid 400 mcg *	Bkfst	Heart	400 mcg	800 mcg	400 mcg
Chromium picolinate 200 mcg	Bkfst Dinner	Diabetes and weight control		400 mcg	400 mcg
Vitamin C 500 mg (Ester C)	Dinner		90 mg	590 mg	700-1000 mg
Vitamin D			400 IU	400 IU	200-400 IU
Vitamin E 400 IU (see EVOLVE) * *	Bkfst	Heart	30 IU	430 IU	600-800 IU
Biotin			30 mcg	30 mcg	under 100
Calcium citrate (200 mg) x 2	Bkfst Dinner	Stones and osteoarthritis	40 mg	440 mg	1 gm
Chloride			7.5 mg	7.5 mg	
Copper			2 mg	2 mg	1.5 -3 mg
Ecotrin (325 mg 4 per wk	Bkfst	Platelets		186 mg	100 mg
Evolve (tocotrienols) 25mg	Dinner	Eendothelium (artery lining)		25 mg	25-50 mg
Iodine			150 mcg	150 mcg	150 mcg
Iron			27 mg	27 mg	10 -15 mg

1 gm = 1,000 mg 1 mg = 1,000 mcg	Individual Pills	Primary purpose	PuritanPride theravim-m	Daily Totals	OPTIMAL
Magnesium oxide 250 mg(150 mg) x 2	Bkfst dinner	Stones & diabetes	100 mg	400 mg	200-400mg
Manganese			5 mg	5 mg	2 -10 mg
Metamucil 1 tsp * * *	lunch			1 tsp	1 tsp
Molybdenum			7.5 mcg	7.5 mcg	50-100mcg
Phosphorus			31 mg	31 mg	
Potassium			7.5 mg	7.5 mg	
SAMe 200 mg X 3	bfst/lun dinner	Depression & osteoarthritis		600 mg	Min. 400 mg
Selenium 100mcg * * * *	bkfst	Heart/prostate	10 mcg	110mcg	100-200mcg
UltraOmega 1 tbsp	lunch	Cardiovascular system		1 tbsp	1 tbsp
Zinc			15 mg	15 mg	15 -30 mg
Claritin 10 mg x 1	bkfst	Pollen		10 mg	10 mg
Asacol 400 mg x 2	bkfst dinner	Colitis & Diverticulosis		800 mg	
Cozaar 50 mg x 1	bkfst	Blood pressure		50 mg	
Glyburide 5 mg x 1	bkfst	Diabetes		5 mg	
Lipitor 20mg x 1 * * * * *	dinner	Lipids & TG		20 mg	
Actos 30 mg x 1	bkfst	Diabetes		30 mg	15 –45 mg

* <u>Folate</u> is all forms of the B vitamin. <u>Folic acid</u> is
synthetic form found only in supplements and fortified
foods.

** Vitamin E <u>SUCCINATE</u> is better than <u>ACETATE</u>. Long-term daily E intake of more than 800 mg can reduce the amounts of A, D, and K that are absorbed from the intestines, possibly causing nausea and diarrhea or even cancer

*** Metamucil should not be taken within two hours of vitamins (could affect body's absorption of certain vitamins)

**** Do not take <u>inorganic</u> selenium at the same time of day as C (C inhibits selenium absorption)

***** Statins (Lipitor) if taken as only one daily dose, should be taken in the evening for best results

7. CONCLUSIONS

The following table (Table 8) shows the results of my four thallium stress tests from early 1990 when my bypass grafts were found to be closing, through December of 1992 when blood flow had been restored to 90% of normal. This is matched against all significant changes affecting my health for the same period. I have taken only the changes from my personal journal (Table 6) that I felt had the most influence on the improved blood flow. Placing each entry within the appropriate calendar quarters was done to provide a more graphic way of assessing time-lapse cause and effect.

Of course, by late 1992 I had managed to keep my cholesterol under 150, my LDL under 100 and my VLDL under 30 virtually 100% of the time for 3 1/2 years. You will recall that these were the target numbers which could bring about a reversal of coronary artery blockage - and that seems to have been

87

exactly what happened, even though it took a few years for those numbers to begin working their magic. As long as I keep these numbers under control and no warning symptoms appear, I see no reason to continue those annual thallium stress tests. Accordingly, I have not had a stress test since 1992.

The medications I have been taking obviously played an important role in bringing those numbers into line, but there were also other factors to consider. During this time, I gradually got to the point where I now stay away from red meat, dairy products, sugar and fried food. Instead, I'm eating lots more fruits and vegetables than I used to. I have also implemented a vitamin/mineral supplementation program that I believe is serving me well.

Another essential element would have to be the less stressful lifestyle I now enjoy. My retirement, coming just when it did, was a real lifesaver, and the resolution of my marital problems was also very important.

Moreover, I am sure that my enthusiastic scampering after tennis balls has been instrumental in causing my body to build a whole new network of natural bypasses to insure that my heart gets an adequate blood supply.

Each part of the battle plan has been helpful, but I am convinced that putting them all together is what tipped the scales in my favor.

TABLE 8 - Cause and effect

Conclusions - using data from table 4 (my blood tests) and table 6 (my journal)				
Qtr	Date	Changes made	Stress test date	Blood flow
1	3/15/90	Began Cardizem SR 180 mg	2/08/90	40%
3	7/23/90	Ecotrin 325mg from 7x weekly to 3x weekly		
4	10/10/90	Marital problems resolved (separated)		

1	2/22/91	Increased Cardizem SR from 180 to 240 mg	2/20/91	60%
3	9/20/91	Began B complex		
4	11/22/91	Began Metamucil (psyllium) 1 tsp daily		

1	1/10/92	Began beta carotene 25,000 IU daily	3/03/92	60%
	3/04/92	From Cardizem SR 240mg to Cardizem CD 300mg		
	3/04/92	From Lovistatin (Mevacor) 40 mg to Zocor 20 mg		
2	6/28/92	Doubled chromium to 400 mg daily		
4	10/20/92	Quit hydrogenated oils	12/22/92	90%

The images showing blood flow to my heart in each of my four thallium stress tests are reproduced below. The jagged area outlined within each circle is the cold spot (where the heart was not getting oxygen at peak exertion). As you can see, the improvement from 1990 to 1992 was dramatic.

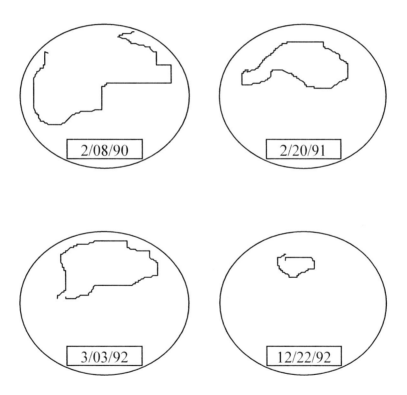

8. INSURANCE CLAIMS

If you have health insurance and/or Medicare, you could drown in a sea of paperwork if you are not organized. Compounding the problem are the frequent errors made by insurance companies in processing and reimbursing their clients' claims. To stay on top of all this, it is essential that you set up a system that will simplify your dealings with your insurer(s). And remember that in all your dealings with health providers and insurers, it is important to make photocopies of anything you mail to them.

I have designed a Medical Claims Worksheet on which to post each expenditure and reimbursement. This worksheet is shown on the next two pages. The first worksheet is blank for you to copy and use as your own. The next page is an example of a completed worksheet. You will notice that there is no column for Medicare. If you are eligible for Medicare, they will be your primary insurer, so use the primary insurer column to post Medicare reimbursements.

Each family member should have two file folders for each health service provider (one for pending claims and one for completed claims). File your worksheets in the appropriate providers' pending folders along with all supporting documents (bills, statements, receipts and EOMB's). When a claim is reimbursed by all your insurers and you have paid the provider, staple all the documents for that claim together and move them from the provider's pending file to the provider's "completed claims" file.

Most doctors automatically submit your Medicare claims for you. If you have a secondary insurer, that insurer may have a working relationship with Medicare (or whoever your primary insurer is) whereby they coordinate your claim benefits between them. In that case, you will not need to submit your claims to either of them. You will be kept informed by means of the Explanation of Medical Benefits

93

Gene McDougall

(EOMB) that your insurers will mail to you. Even so, I urge you to post those transactions on your worksheet so you can easily keep track of the paperwork.

Having a record of all your medical expenses and reimbursements as well as photocopies of all the documents involved will come in handy when you find it necessary to contact your insurance company to point out errors they have made. Yes, they will make errors from time to time, but if you keep records and stay organized, most problems can be resolved quite easily.

_____'s MEDICAL CLAIM WORKSHEET FOR PROVIDER _____

SERVICE	DATE	COST	AMOUNT PAID BY PRIMARY INSURER (EOMB RECEIVED)	AMOUNT PAID BY SECONDARY INSURER (EOMB RECEIVED)	AMOUNT I OWE TO PROVIDER	DATE I PAID PROVIDER (PAY PROVIDER ONLY AFTER RECEIVING EOMB'S FROM BOTH INSURERS)

GENE 's MEDICAL CLAIM WORKSHEET FOR PROVIDER DR. MCDUFF

SERVICE	DATE	COST	AMOUNT PAID BY PRIMARY INSURER (EOMB RECEIVED)	AMOUNT PAID BY SECONDARY INSURER (EOMB RECEIVED)	AMOUNT I OWE TO PROVIDER	DATE I PAID PROVIDER (PAY PROVIDER ONLY AFTER RECEIVING EOMB'S FROM BOTH INSURERS)
VISIT	8/20/00	32.00	25.60	3.20	3.22	12/22/00
XRAYS	9/08/00	119.25	95.40	23.85	11.92	1/10/01

EPILOGUE

Since I am not a doctor, I would not presume to give medical advice to anyone. I can only pass along my own experiences and offer my own assumptions regarding what may have contributed to my increased blood flow and general good health.

It is up to you to decide for yourself what to take from all this, just as I had to decide what path was best for me as I collected and evaluated tons of sometimes contradictory information from hundreds of sources.

I hope what I have shared with you will be useful. I can think of no better way to conclude than by quoting a wonderful paragraph from Norman Cousins' book, "Head First". To me, these words are sheer poetry:

"The evidence is mounting that the heart can make its own bypass under circumstances of arterial blockage. Narrowing of the heart's arteries can be caused by a diet heavy in fats and cholesterol and by a life-style high in stress and low in exercise. But the elimination of these faults can sometimes produce a natural bypass in which the heart receives an augmented supply of oxygen through a rich new network of blood vessels. Heart attack sufferers who are able to apply themselves diligently to a new life-style stand a good chance of reaping these benefits."

ABOUT THE AUTHOR

Gene McDougall has survived a rebellious youth, two high school stabbings, two automobile rollover accidents (yes, being a teenager was dangerous even in circa 1945 small-town Minnesota), a four-year hitch in the Navy, 28 months of which was spent as a prisoner on Guam (he says he was held there against his will when the Navy refused to grant his transfer request), four years at the University of Minnesota earning his BA in Journalism, a 31-year ordeal in the corporate jungle (from which he emerged not only unscathed, but with a vice presidency), three spinal surgeries, one heart attack and one quintuple heart bypass operation. Needless to say, his sense of humor has also survived intact.

Since his retirement in 1987, he has been enjoying what he happily describes as the best days of his life. He makes his home in Arlington Heights, a pleasant suburb northwest of Chicago where he has resided since 1970. He plays a strenuous hour or two of singles tennis three days a week and spends the rest of his time watching television, reading and pursuing his first love, writing.

He has co-authored one previous book, "Cow Pies, A Messy Journey Through The Pasture of Life" with his good friend, Nelson Campbell, and he is currently working on a third book - "Letters to David Letterman."

Printed in the United States
21251LVS00001B/11-12